Faustin Kamuanga Kapaza
Jean Félix Kabangu Ngoyi
Freddy Munung Nguej

HIV/AIDS Prevention and Health Promotion

Faustin Kamuanga Kapaza
Jean Félix Kabangu Ngoyi
Freddy Munung Nguej

HIV/AIDS Prevention and Health Promotion

Explanatory factors for the low use of VCT by the population aged 15 years and over. (Case of the town of Mwene-Ditu in DR Congo)

ScienciaScripts

Explanatory factors for the low use of VCT by the population aged 15 years and over (case of the town of Mwene-Ditu in DR Congo).

By KAMUANGA KAPAZA Faustin1, KABANGU NGOYI Jean Félix2 and MUNUNG NGUEJ Freddy3

SUMMARY

HIV infection is currently one of the leading causes of mortality and morbidity in countries around the world, the Democratic Republic of Congo in general and the town of Mwene-Ditu in particular are no exception. Ignorance of HIV status is a major factor in the spread of the disease. For this reason, we conducted a descriptive and cross-sectional observational study from 15 June to 15 July 2020, i.e. one month in our railway town of Mwene-Ditu. It consisted in identifying not only the explanatory factors of low utilization of voluntary HIV counselling and testing services (VCT), but also in determining the socio-demographic characteristics of the users of this service. The usual descriptive and epidemiological statistical analyses were carried out for this purpose to determine the associations between certain variables studied.

At the end of our survey, 333 statistical units were interviewed and the findings from these interviews showed a predominance of people who did not know their HIV status 86% against only 14% who knew their HIV status and who said they had used VCT at least once. This low use was significantly linked to certain factors, namely age under 30 years, i.e. 15-25 years (OR=0.24 [0.11-0.50]); the occupation category "hobbyist" (OR= 0.15[0.04-0.56]); the level of primary education (OR= 0.08[0.02-0.30]); ignorance of the place of screening (OR= 0.21[0.07-0.59]); lack of awareness (OR= 0.16[0.07-0.38]). These results show the need to continue to intensify sensitisation to encourage and orient the population to use the VCT service, which contributes effectively to the prevention and reduction of new HIV infections in the population.

Keywords: Factors, Explanatory, Low utilization, VCT, Population.

[1] KAMUANGA KAPAZA Faustin: Assistant at the University of Mwene-Ditu in Public Health ;
[2] KABANGU NGOYI Jean Félix: Assistant at the University of Mwene-Ditu in Public Health;
[3] MUNUNG NGUEJ Freddy: Assistant2 at the Higher Institute of Medical Techniques, ISTM Musumba.

INTRODUCTION

1. Statement of the problem

HIV, a retrovirus that primarily affects T4 lymphocytes, is the causative agent of acquired immunodeficiency syndrome (AIDS). Testing for this condition can either be done at a health facility or at a voluntary testing centre (VCT).

VCT services contribute to the prevention of HIV infection. They are a right of every individual. The universal ambition is that by the year 2020, at least 90% of infected people know their HIV status (UNAIDS, 2015). This is an ambitious goal, but it must be achieved in accordance with ethical principles (WHO, 2015).

HIV/AIDS is now one of the diseases responsible for high mortality and morbidity in the world. From the beginning of the epidemic until 2018, 32 million people have died. In addition, it is increasingly affecting young people (UNAIDS, 2019).

According to the UNAIDS report 2018 (2019), there were 37.9 million adults living with HIV; 1.7 million children under 15 years of age and 770,000 AIDS-related deaths worldwide. Many infants and children infected with HIV were dying of HIV-related causes without knowing their HIV status and without receiving adequate care (WHO, 2008).

HIV/AIDS is one of the most devastating communicable diseases of the last three decades. Its impact in resource-constrained countries is significant. Consequences include large numbers of deaths, especially of mothers and children; reduced economic productivity in countries where high prevalence persists; increased fragility of health systems; and social disruption. (WHO, 2019).

The 24 countries that make up the West and Central Africa region are home to 25% of children aged 0-14 years and 16% of adults among PLWHA worldwide. Among these countries, Nigeria has the highest rate (49%), followed by Cameroon, Côte d'Ivoire and Ghana. DR Congo has the second highest proportion of children living with HIV, at 9% (UNICEF/UNAIDS; 2017).

According to a study conducted in Cameroon by Mbompi-Keou et al. (2013), the prevalence of HIV infection was 2.6%. It was 3 times higher among women.

The DRC has a generalised epidemic with an average prevalence of 1.2% in the general population and 2.1% among pregnant women (PNLS, 2017). According to the PNMLS (2018), the prevalence of HIV infection was estimated to be 0.9% and 3.3% and 1.7% and 2.46% respectively in the town of Kabinda and the town of Mwene-Ditu in

Lomami province.

By 2030, it will be time for the evaluation of the MDGs, in which one of the major objectives related to the fight against HIV is the proportion of people who know their HIV status, which must be 90%. However, epidemiological data show that there is still a significant proportion of people who do not know their status for various reasons (WHO, 2016). In order to increase the proportion of people who know their serological status, strategies have been put in place including self-testing, VCT, DCIP, PMTCT etc. (PNMLS, 2018)

For Kitahata et al. (2009) and Rozenbaum (2010), ignorance of HIV status is an important factor in the spread of the disease. Hence, testing remains the gateway to HIV prevention (Memmi et al., 2010). Therefore, it is important to use all strategies to increase the proportion of people who know their HIV status.

The following questions will be answered in some way during the course of our research:

- What are the socio-demographic characteristics of VCT users?

- What are the factors that explain the low use of VCT services by the interviewed population?

In view of the morbidity and mortality of HIV infection, it goes without saying that the study on knowledge of one's serological status is relevant. In addition, the United Nations 9090-90 objectives require an intensification of actions to identify people with the virus and to take care of them early. In relation to the first 90, the supply and demand for VCT services remains unavoidable.

The observation is that the population's use of VCT is low. However, in our environment, there are no studies on the factors explaining the low use of VCT. The available studies have dealt with women undergoing PMTCT and the screening of children under 15 years of age. This is what prompted us to address this topic.

2. Review of the literature

Globally, according to UNAIDS (2019), 79% [67-92%] of all people living with HIV know their HIV status.

In France, 5.03 million HIV serological tests were performed; this represented an 8% proportion of people who knew their serological status. (Girard et al., 2008).

In the United States, according to Marks' study in 2005 and 2006, knowledge of HIV status reduced the annual number of new HIV infections from sexual transmission by 31%.

In Africa, an estimated 36% of PLHIV were aware of their HIV status in the western and central part of the continent compared to 56% in the southern and eastern part (UNAIDS, 2016).

In Botswana, it has been shown that sexually active young people do not want to be tested for HIV; this is a barrier to improved testing (Fako, 2006).

In the South African region, knowledge of HIV was a prerequisite for requesting the test. (Fylkesnes et al, 2004; Degraft et al, 2005, Peltzer et al, 2009).

In Burkina Faso, studies have shown good acceptance of HIV testing by pregnant women (Sarker et al., 2009). In a multivariate analysis of repeat VCT use, an association between seronegativity and schooling but also young age was noted (Rouamba, 2016). (Rouamba, 2016).

In 2014, it was shown that about 50% of the population had access to serological testing (Somé et al., 2014). Although there was an increase in the offer of VCT to pregnant women to 86% at the first ANC visit, a small proportion returned for results (Somé et al., 2015).

According to studies by Peltzer (2009) and Snow (2010), women had more access to VCT than men. Women accounted for 65% of those tested. In contrast, Hutchinson (2006) showed in his study that men in relationships were more likely to test for HIV. People aged 25 and over were more likely to know their HIV status than younger people (Peltzer et al., 2009; Jhonston et al., 2010).

In Togo, family-based testing has proven to be one of the most effective and cost-effective ways to identify children living with HIV. (Singo et al., 2016).

An in-depth analysis of the triple 90 shows that countries in West and Central Africa, including DRC, lag behind other countries (WHO, 2019). There are several plausible causes for the 1:90. Studies conducted to find out the reasons for not knowing HIV status have found fear of HIV-positive status as a fundamental barrier (Meiberg et al., 2008; Mutalemwa et al., 2008; Kranzer et al., 2008; Osinde et al., 2011).

According to Neuman et al. (2013), rates of HIV-related stigma in interpersonal relationships were highest in Malawi and Burkina Faso at 43% and 40% respectively.

In Uganda, an analysis from 2008 to 2009 showed that men were not using HIV testing services because of stigma (Larsson et al., 2010). In South Africa, potential barriers to receiving or providing HIV testing included 16.4% of patients and 24% of providers stating that the subject of HIV was too sensitive and 58.7% of patients and 80% of providers stating that privacy and confidentiality were violated (Hansoti et al., 2017).

Fear of stigma leads to fear and reluctance to test for HIV (Meiberg et al., 2008; Makhlouf et al., 2009; Maman et al., 2009). In the study by Pulerwitz (2010), it was shown that despite the widespread stigma of HIV, it is possible to implement programmes that help reduce it among health workers, service providers and the public.

Barriers to adolescents' access to HIV testing include age of consent laws and parental consent requirements, fear of stigma, reactions of relatives etc. (Agudu et al., 2016).

According to Desclaux (2014), the limitations of knowing one's HIV status were related to crowding or the fear of not being supported in case of a positive result.

Negative reactions result in low levels of sharing of HIV status, especially with partners; this does not encourage couple testing (Mutalemwa et al., 2008; Maman et al., 2009).

In the Democratic Republic of Congo, HIV testing rates were estimated at 26.6% with an estimated seropositivity of 2.2%. The said seroprevalence was higher among pregnant women at 9.9% (PNLS, 2018). According to a study conducted in Lubumbashi, a high prevalence of HIV was observed among children, thus justifying the need to carry out VCT among parents (Tshikwej et al., 2017).

The study by Tshikwej (2015) showed that the risk of mother-to-child transmission of HIV infection was significantly associated with factors such as testing at delivery or during breastfeeding.

According to Mwembo (2012), low education and ignorance of vertical transmission of HIV were the factors determining ignorance of HIV status among women.

According to the NMCP (2019), HIV testing rates vary from province to province. It was 48.8% in Equateur; in Kasai province 52.1%; in Kasai centrale, 33.5%; in Kasai oriental, 47.3% and in the city province of Kinshasa, 69.2% etc. In Lomami province, the 2018 epidemiological data had indicated that 12,797 people were sensitised and the rate of testing was 15.8%.

In 2019, according to the PNLS Lomami BPC, 510,063 people were counselled at the VCT of which 17,205 cases were tested for HIV, representing 3.37% of the test completion rate.

3. Objectives

3.1. General objective

The overall objective of this study is to contribute to the reduction of morbidity and mortality due to HIV infection by improving access to VCT for the population aged 15 years and over.

3.2. Specific objectives

- Describe or identify the socio-demographic characteristics of VCT users;
- To determine the factors underlying low utilization of VCT services by the population aged 15 years and over.

4. Assumptions

Factors for low uptake of VCT services for the population aged 15 years and above in the railway town of Mwene-Ditu in the province of Lomami would be: gender, level of education, occupation, religion, fear of positive results, fear of HIV-related stigma, age, lack of knowledge about VCT and HIV services.

Chapter 1

GENERAL INFORMATION ON HIV INFECTION

1.1. Historical overview

AIDS first appeared in the 1950s in Africa, but these few sporadic cases went unnoticed. The first groups of patients sufficient to define the new syndrome were identified in California and New York in 1981. Two years later, the viral origin of the condition and its main modes of transmission were known. From then on, what seemed to be an epidemic affecting the American homosexual population became one of the most serious pandemics of the 21st century.

1.2. Definition

HIV infection is a disease caused by HIV, which is characterised by the invasion of immune cells, particularly CD4 cells.

AIDS (Acquired Immune Deficiency Syndrome) is a chronic infection that is caused by the destruction of the immune system by a virus called HIV (Human Immunodeficiency Virus).

1.3. Etiopathogenesis

1.3.1. Types of HIV

Currently, there are two types of virus in circulation. These are HIV-1 and HIV-2. Both viruses eventually lead to the same disease, but HIV-2 is less virulent and its progression to AIDS is slower. HIV-1 is the most circulating type in the world and the most common in the DRC.

1.3.2. Transmission routes

There are three routes of transmission of HIV infection:

- **Sexual:** Most frequent in Africa (80-90%), due to unprotected vaginal, anal and oral sex.

- **The blood route:** Represents 5 to 10% of contamination routes. It occurs through the transfusion of HIV-contaminated blood (with a 98% probability of infection) and the use of soiled sharp objects.

- **The vertical route (from mother to child):** variable between 30% and 40%, during pregnancy, childbirth and breastfeeding.

1.3.3. Risk and non-risk factors

Several risk factors are involved in the spread of HIV infection:

- Biological or medical factors: rape, untested blood transfusions, fellatio etc. ;

- Social cultural factors: sorority ;

- Social demographic factors: population movement, promiscuity etc;

- Social economic factors: poverty, sharing of sharps etc;

- Psychological factors: curiosity etc.

Safe factors include: insect bites, kissing, hugging, exchanging cloths, sharing food, washing dishes etc. (WHO, 2017)

1.3.4. Exposed groups and risk behaviours

- The groups exposed include:

Homosexuals, heterosexuals, drug users, haemophiliacs, blood recipients, people with multiple and occasional partners, newborns of HIV-positive mothers, medical and paramedical staff.

- Risk behaviours include:

Unprotected anal or vaginal penetration; sharing needles, syringes, other injection equipment or contaminated solutions when injecting drugs; injections; unsafe blood transfusions; medical procedures that involve cutting or piercing the skin under unsterile conditions; and accidental needle sticks, especially among health workers. (WHO, 2017).

1.4. Stages of HIV

There are four (4) phases of HIV infection, which are

1.4.1. Phase 1: Primary infection

In the weeks (2-3) following infection, flu-like symptoms may occur in 20-30% of those infected.

1.4.2. Phase 2: asymptomatic

This period of time is called the "window period" during which the person tests negative although the virus is present and multiplying.

Seroconversion is when antibodies to HIV become detectable in the blood.

1.4.3. Phase 3: symptomatic

This is the longest phase. There are no clinical manifestations but sometimes persistent generalised lymphadenopathy or progressive deterioration of CD4 lymphocytes.

It is characterised by the appearance of various clinical manifestations such as weight loss, prolonged fevers, chronic diarrhoea, generalised dermatitis, etc.

1.4.4. Phase 4: AIDS

This phase can take 2 to 15 years to appear, depending on the case. It is characterised by an advanced breakdown of the immune system, opening the way for opportunistic infections.

1.5. Screening concepts

According to the NMCP (2019), HIV testing rates vary from province to province. It was 48.8% in Equateur; in Kasai province 52.1%; in Kasai centrale, 33.5%; in Kasai oriental, 47.3% and in the city province of Kinshasa, 69.2% etc. In Lomami province, the 2018 epidemiological data had indicated that 12,797 people were sensitised and the rate of testing was 15.8%.

In 2019, according to the PNLS Lomami BPC, 510,063 people were counselled at the VCT of which 17,205 cases were tested for HIV, representing 3.37% of the test completion rate.

1.5.1. Type of screening

There are various types of screening, each with a specific purpose:

- Mass screening which covers a large number of the population;

- Multiphase screening, which uses a number of tests on the same occasion;

- Targeted screening of groups with particular exposures is often used in the context of environmental and occupational health;

- Proactive or systematic screening: population registers are used to invite members of a population at risk to be screened at appropriate intervals;

- Case finding or opportunistic screening is a form of screening that is limited to patients who consult a health professional for another purpose.

- Voluntary testing is when a person voluntarily gets tested in order to find out their HIV status.

1.5.2. The Principles of Screening

The five recommended principles include

- Informed consent ;

- Confidentiality ;

- The board;

- Accuracy of screening results ;

- Linking to care and treatment services (WHO, 2019).

1.5.3. Steps in screening advice

Several stages are identified in the conduct of screening, namely

- Pre-test counselling which seeks informed consent to HIV testing and preparation for the announcement of the test result;

- The performance of the test (sampling and analysis) that allows the biological diagnosis of HIV infection;

- Post-test counselling, which includes the announcement of the result, psychosocial management of the client's reaction and prevention counselling.

If positive, referral to a biomedical and psychological care network is required.

1.5.4. Role of a VCT

VCT is a voluntary HIV counselling and testing service that enables individuals to find out their HIV status. It plays an important role in the prevention of HIV infection.

In addition, it facilitates the early and appropriate use of services by HIV-positive and HIV-negative people, such as care, family planning, psychological and social support or counselling, legal assistance and positive living advice (UNAIDS, 2019).

Chapter 2

WAYS TO PREVENT HIV INFECTION

Prevention of HIV infection remains one of the effective strategies to control and eliminate this disease as a public health problem in the world in general and in the most affected countries in particular. Thus, there are several means of prevention.

2.1. Prevention methods

They are closely related to the modes or routes of HIV infection and can be summarised in three:

2.1.1. Prevention of sexual transmission

This prevention can be summarised in strategies known as A B C, i.e:

- Abstinence,

- Good loyalty,

- Condom use: The consistent and correct use of male or female condoms during all sexual encounters between partners.

2.1.2. Prevention of blood-borne transmission

In this group, we can mention :

- Transfusion safety: Bringing blood banks up to international standards and respecting these standards; transfusing only when strictly necessary, blood must be tested for four (4) markers before being transfused;

- Intramuscular and intravenous injection with sterilised and single-use equipment;

- Use single-use equipment whenever necessary, including for certain practices such as circumcision;

- Avoid injuries from soiled sharps. In case of injury, disinfect as soon as possible.

2.1.2. Prevention of mother-to-child transmission (PMTCT)

With regard to this transmission, it requires strong mobilisation and awareness-raising on the risks of vertical transmission of HIV from mother to child. This prevention uses four major components (pillars) of PMTCT, as follows

- Prevention of HIV infection in women of childbearing age ;

- Prevention of unintended pregnancies in HIV-infected women ;

- Prevention of HIV transmission from an HIV-infected woman to her baby ;

- Provides care and support to HIV-infected women, their babies and their families (NMCP, 2017).

2.2. Combined prevention

It consists of both pre- and post-exposure prophylaxis:

2.2.1. Pre-exposure prophylaxis (PrEP)

This is the use of antiretroviral treatment to prevent HIV infection in HIV-negative people at substantial risk of contracting HIV, in DR Congo this includes

- Discordant couples ;
- Gender professionals ;
- Men who have sex with men (MSM) ;
- Injecting drug users (IDUs) ;
- Transgender.

PrEP must necessarily be started as soon as a person tests negative for HIV. The recipient will need to be prepared to have continuous follow-up with HIV tests every three months. This practice will continue to be administered as long as exposure exists (NACP, 2017).

2.2.2. Post-exposure prophylaxis (PEP)

It is the administration of therapeutic agents to prevent infection after exposure to a pathogen. This PEP covers prevention of HIV, STIs, hepatitis and pregnancy. In all cases, psychosocial support is essential for trauma management and treatment adherence. Two types of risk are distinguished in this prophylaxis: accidental exposure to blood or body fluids and sexual exposure (NACP, 2017).

This intervention consists of ARV treatment within 28 days. It is offered and administered to all people who have had an exposure that could result in HIV transmission, ideally within 72 hours. Practising this prevention can reduce the risk of HIV infection by more than 80%.

Furthermore, rapid access to PEP remains difficult in many settings, especially when it is not a health worker (Anon, 2014).

2.3. Benefits associated with HIV testing

Motivations for screening correspond to an individual's desire to find out his or her serological status. However, two main objectives can be assigned to screening for HIV infection:

- At the individual level, to enable the early implementation of therapeutic or prophylactic interventions in order to reduce morbidity and mortality (for HIV-positive people) and to encourage preventive behaviour for HIV-negative people;
- At the collective level, limit the spread of the epidemic by empowering people

living with HIV to change their risky practices and by reducing the transmission of those on treatment.

These general objectives fall under both primary and secondary prevention.

Screening could reduce HIV transmission rates in two ways:

- Directly through a reduction in risky practices;

- Indirectly through the identification of additional infected persons who meet the criteria for initiation of HAART, which in turn leads to a reduction in infection among infected persons.

2.4. Ethical aspects of routine screening

Expanding HIV testing as a precondition for improving access to treatment must be based on: respect, protection and fulfilment of human rights standards.

Voluntary testing must remain at the heart of all HIV policies and programmes to respect human rights principles and to ensure sustainable public health benefits (PHAC, 2006).

Chapter 3

METHODS

3.1. Research framework

This study was conducted in the town of Mwene-Ditu, located in the province of LOMAMI in DR Congo. It comprises three communes (Bondoyi, Musadi and Mwene-Ditu) and two health zones (Makota and Mwene-Ditu).

It has an estimated population of 1,278,789, of which the commune of Bondoyi has an estimated population of 422,558, Musadi 385,120 and Mwene- Ditu 471,111.

3.1.1. General Information

The town of Mwene-Ditu contains the different tribes namely: Kanyok, Kete, Luba, Songe etc. The main activities of the population of this town are: agriculture, small businesses, cattle and poultry breeding.

3.2. Operational definitions of the concepts used

- **Use**: Action, way of using; employment, it is the way or manner in which the VCT is used/frequented by the population under study;

- **Service**: is a place where health care is administered. It is the place where not only the voluntary HIV test is carried out, but also the counselling given to the service users before and after the test;

- **Population**: this is the totality of people living in a given environment, in the context of our research it is the inhabitants of the town of Mwene-Ditu as a whole;

- **Screening**: According to the World Health Organization (2016), screening is the presumptive identification of individuals with a previously undetected disease or abnormality through the use of systematic and standardised tests;

- **VCT**: is a set of services that are offered to populations to give them the opportunity to know their HIV status based on an informed decision;

- **HIV: is** a retrovirus that primarily affects T4 lymphocytes and is the causative agent of Acquired Immunodeficiency Syndrome (AIDS).

3.3. Type of study

We conducted a cross-sectional observational study with an analytical and monocentric aim. It took place over a period of one month, from 15 June to 15 July 2020.

3.4. Population: statistical units

The source or target population was people living in the town of Mwene-Ditu. The population aged 15 years and above, being the sexually active population at risk of HIV infection, was the target population for our study.

3.5. Sampling method

3.5.1. *Selection criteria*

- *Inclusion criteria*: all residents of Mwene-Ditu aged 15 years and over who gave their free consent to participate in this survey were included in our sample.

- *Exclusion criteria*: Any person who refused to answer certain questions during the course of the survey was automatically excluded from the study.

3.5.2. *Sampling*

In relation to the sampling technique, we used several methods to identify the statistical units to be included in our study as follows:

In the first stage, non-probability convenience sampling was used to select all three communes that make up the town of Mwene-Ditu (Bondoyi, Musadi and Mwene-Ditu);

In the second stage, stratified random sampling was adopted. The stratification was done on the basis of households;

- At the first level, we randomly selected 3 neighbourhoods in each commune, which allowed us to retain 9 neighbourhoods in which to conduct our survey;

- At the second level, in each district we selected 3 cells. Thus, the total number of cells selected for this study was 27;

- At the third level, we selected two avenues at random and in each avenue two households were selected in a systematic and simple way. Placed in the middle of the avenue, the interviewer threw a pen in the air and the orientation of the ball determined the first household to be surveyed. Then the sampling step was determined by the formula below and followed to identify the [second] household to be surveyed:

K = With:

- K: no survey

- N: number of households per avenue

- n: number of units to be surveyed (5 households).

Beforehand, a quota for each municipality was determined in order to reach our sample size. This was determined by the following formula:

With:

- n= size of statistical units to be surveyed within the municipality (quota) ;

- N= total sample size ;

n=

All adults found in the households identified as described above who had given their consent were interviewed until the quota for each commune was reached to obtain our total sample size.

3.5.3. Sample size

The minimum sample size was calculated using the SHWATZ formula below considering the 27% HIV test completion rate reported at the national level in the report (NMCP, 2018):

n=

With:

- n: sample size ;
- Z: reduced deviation, statistical table value at 5% = 1.96 ;
- P: percentage of test completion;
- d: risk of error or margin of error at 5%.

Given that:

P=27% = 0.27; q: 1-0.27=0.73, taking Z (95%)=1.96 and d (5%)=0.05; the size should be :

$$n = \frac{(1.96)^2 \, X \, 0.27 \, X \, 0.733}{(0,05)^{2=0}} \quad \frac{.8416 \, X \, 0.730}{,0025=0} \quad \frac{.75717936}{,0025} = 302{,}87 \sim 303$$

Taking into account the proportion of non-respondents, the adjustment consisted in adding 10% of the size to the value obtained. The final adjusted sample size was 333 statistical units.

3.6. Method of data collection

In order to collect useful information for this study, a semi-structured questionnaire was designed for this purpose and pre-tested in the commune of Mwene-Ditu in the Kabila Kabange district to obtain certain reactions before our actual survey in order to adjust and improve certain questions in relation to the reactions observed in the field.

After determining the neighbourhoods, the cells on paper based on the sampling methods mentioned above, we went out into the field to identify the households in which we interviewed people aged 15 and over who had agreed to participate in this study.

3.7. Data management and statistical analysis

The collected data were encoded on Excel (Microsoft, 2007) and then imported for processing on Epi Info 7.2.2.6 (CDC, 2016). The results were presented in the form of tables and figures with the observed numbers, proportions with their 95% confidence intervals and the parameters of central tendency (means and medians) and dispersions (minimum, maximum and standard deviation).

The epidemiological parameters Odds ratio (OR) and Chi-square were used to establish the relationships between our variables and even check their strengths.

Links were significant when the OR was greater than 1 with the lower bound also greater than 1 (95% CI).

Whenever the OR was less than 1 and its upper bound less than 1 (95% CI), there was no association between the associated variables. But in the context of our study as we are dealing with the factors that explain the low use of VCT, the significant association of OR less than 1 is considered in its negative sense than in its positive sense mentioned above when it comes to studying the association of a morbid phenomenon where it is considered a protective factor. In our study, when the OR was less than 1 and its upper limit less than 1, this association was considered statistically significant while verifying its significance with the small p less than 0.05. Thus, the Chi-square was significant when it was greater than 3.84 at the degree of freedom (ddl) which is equal to 1.

3.8. Ethical considerations

When we went to the field to make contact with the interviewees, confidentiality was not only guaranteed, but also respected, and a written informed consent was signed for our protection.

Chapter 4

RESULTS

The study sample consisted of 333 respondents from three communes in the city of Mwene-Ditu. Each commune was represented by a quota determined according to the method described above.

After data collection and analysis, the results are as follows:

4.1. Socio-demographic characteristics

Table I: Distribution of respondents by age

Age range (years)	Frequency	%	95% CI
[15-25[	172	51,7%	[46,1-57,1]
[25-35[	86	25,8%	[21,3-30,9]
[35-45[	33	9,9%	[7-13,8]
[45-55[	20	6,0%	[3,8-9,3]
[55-65[	12	3,6%	[2-6,4]
[65-75[	9	2,7%	[1,3-5,2]
[75-85[	1	0,3%	[0-1,9]
Total	**333**	**100**	

Table I shows that respondents in the 15-25 age group accounted for more than half of the total sample 51.7% [95% CI; 46.1-57.1] and those in the 75-85 age group accounted for only 0.3% [95% CI; 0-1.9].

Table II. Age distribution parameters

Parameters	Value
Minimum and maximum	15-82 years
Average	28.6 (Sdv 13.3%)
Median	24 years old
Mode	18 years old
First quartile	19 years old
Third quartile	34 years old

From the above table it can be seen that the minimum age of our respondents was 15 years and the maximum was 82 years, giving an average age of 28.6 (Sdv 13.3).

From Figure 1 below, it can be seen that females accounted for 51% [95% CI 45.8-56.8] and males for 49% [95% CI 43.2- 54.2].

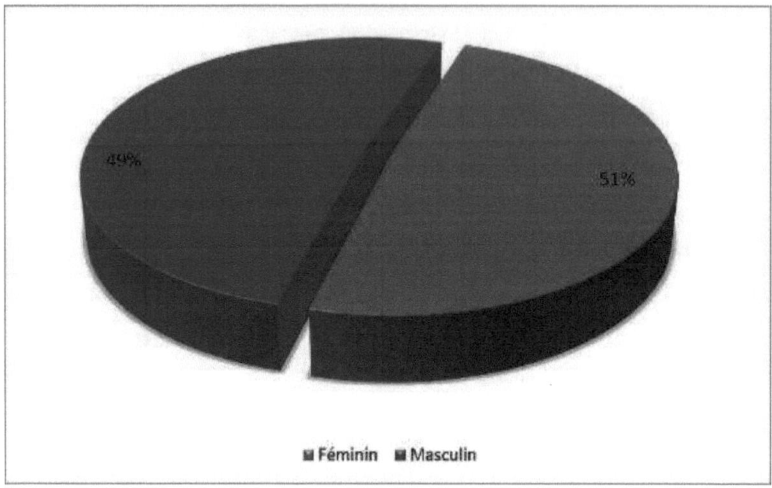

Fig.1: Distribution of respondents by gender.

According to the results in the figure below, students accounted for 28.8% [95% CI 24.1- 34.1] and professionals for 3% [95% CI 1.5% - 5.6] of the respondents.

Distribution by occupation

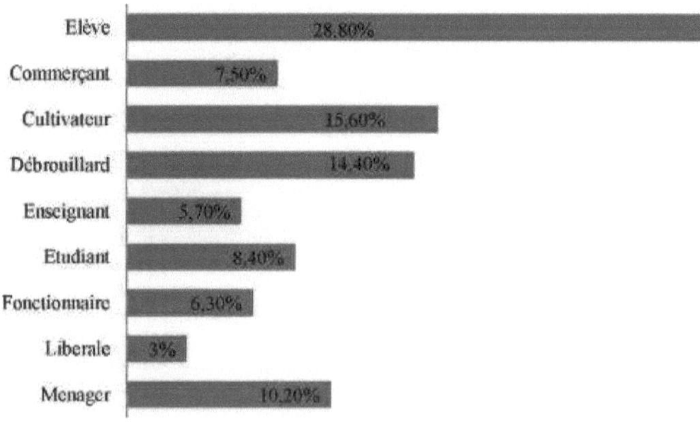

Fig. 2: Distribution of respondents by occupation

According to Figure 3 below, 54% [95% CI 48.2-59.2] of respondents were single and 2% [95% CI 1.1-4.9] were widowed.

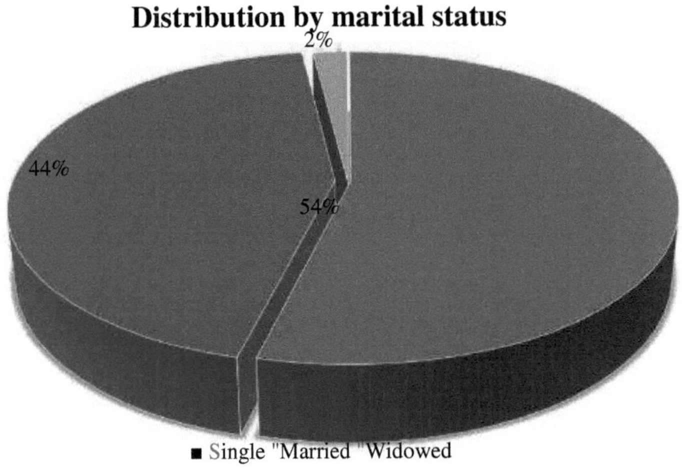

Fig. 3: Distribution of respondents by marital status.

Figure 4 shows that primary education accounted for 44% [95% CI 38.249.1] of respondents and those with no education for 3% [95% CI 1.7-6].

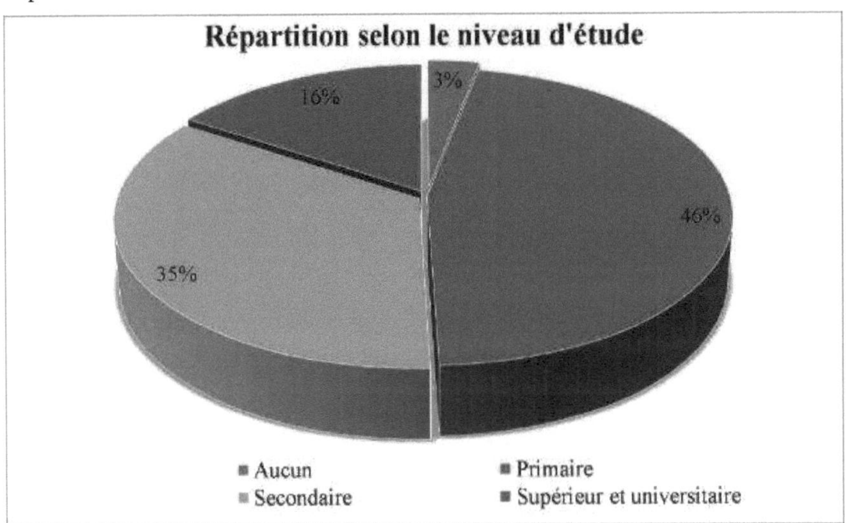

Fig.4: Distribution of respondents by level of education

The data presented in Figure 5 shows that Christians accounted for 89% [95% CI 85-92.1] and animists 1% [95% CI 0.2-2.8].

Distribution by religion

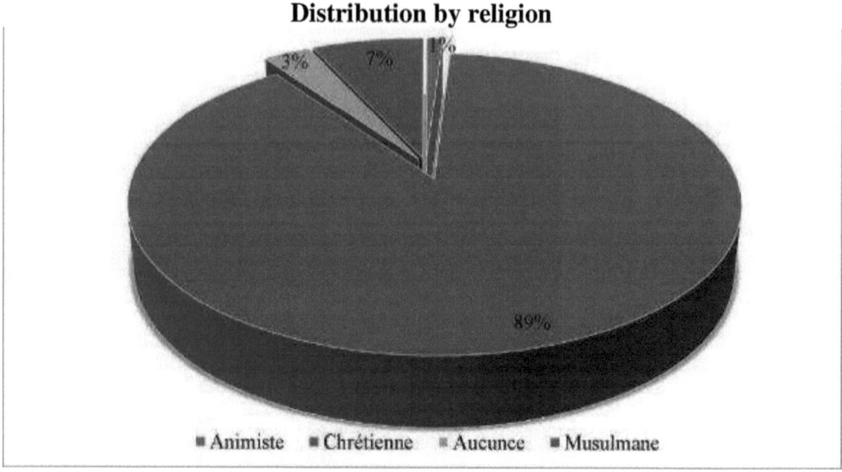

Fig. 5: Distribution of cases by religion

From Figure 6, we see that 37% [95% CI 31.8-42.4] of respondents resided in the commune of Mwene-Ditu, and 30% [95% CI 25.2-35.3] in the commune of Musadi.

Distribution by residence

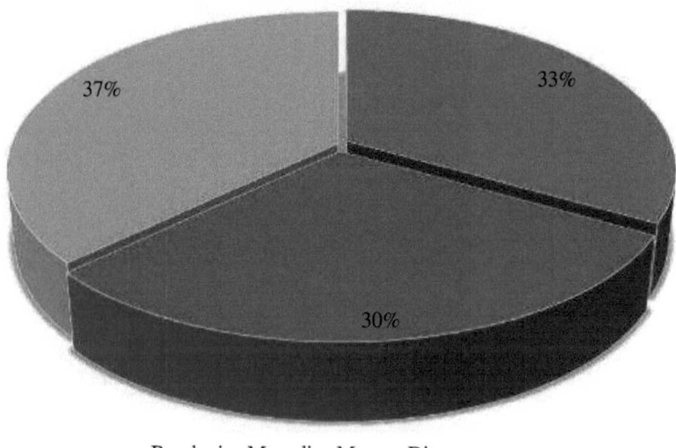

Fig. 6: Distribution of interviewees by residence.

The results in Figure 7 show that 86% [95% CI 82-89.7] of respondents did not know their HIV status and 14% [95% CI 10.4-18.1] knew their HIV status.

Distribution according to knowledge of serological status

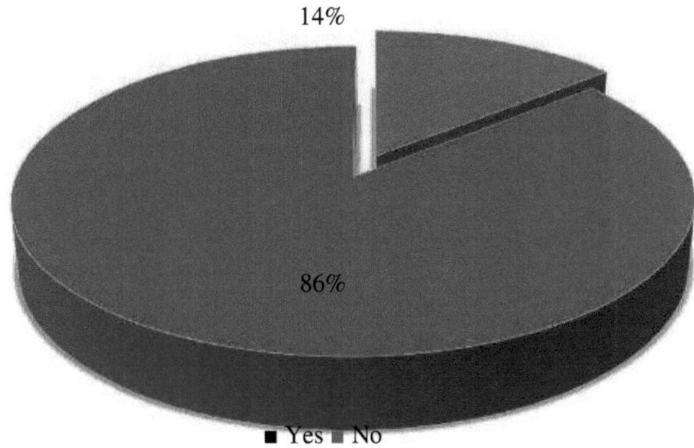

Fig. 7: Distribution of cases by knowledge of HIV status

According to Figure 8, 52% [95% CI 45.6-57.5] of the respondents agreed to have the HIV test done later and 48% [95% CI 42.5-54.4] refused.

Répartition selon l'avis accordé au test

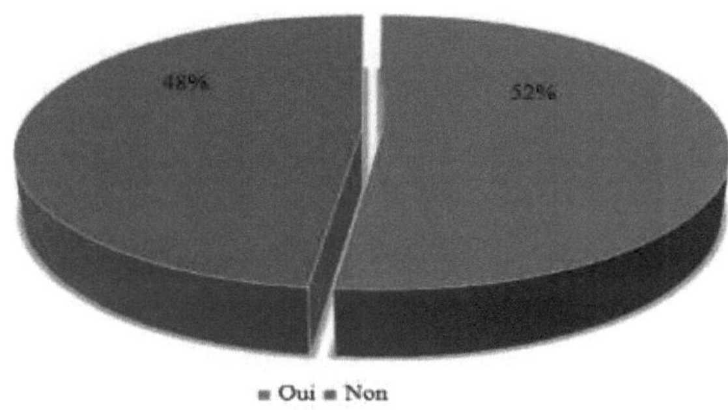

The data in the figure below shows that 30% [95% CI 22.738.6] of respondents

Fig.8: Distribution of ca's according to their opinion on the HIV test

refused to take the test because of discrimination and 19% [95% CI 13.2-27] because of provider discretion or non-confidentiality.

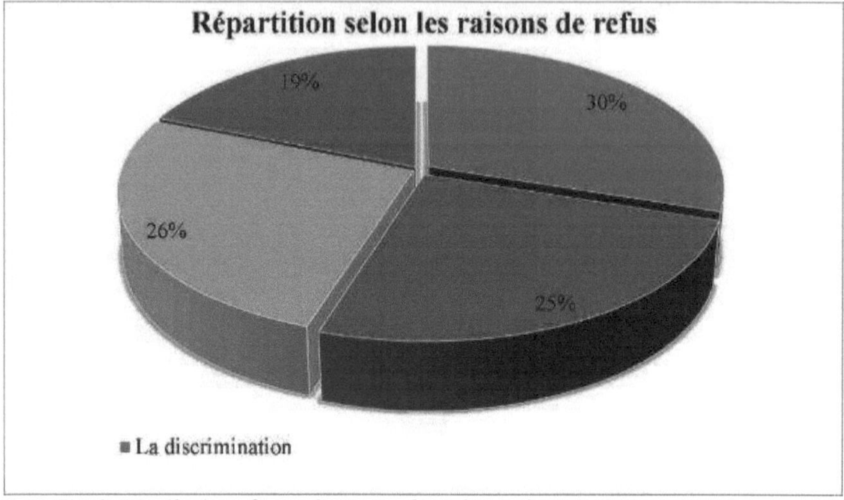

Fig. 9: Distribution of cases by reason for refusal of HIV testing

4.2. Associations of variables

4.2.1. Associations between socio-demographic characteristics and the use of HIV voluntary counselling and testing (VCT) service

Table III. Gender and VCT use

Gender	Use of VCT		Total	OR [95% CI]	x2	p-value
	Yes	No				
Female	24(14)	147(86)	171	Reference		
male	22(13,6)	140(86,4)	162	0,96[0,51-1,79]	0,001	1
Total	**46**	**287**	**333**			

The above contingency table shows that there is no statistically significant association between the gender of the respondents and low VCT use. OR=0.96 [0.51-1.79], **x2** less than 3.84 at ddl= 1 and P-value greater than 0.05.

Table IV. Age and VCT use

Age groups (years)	Use of VCT		Total	OR [95% CI]	x2	p-value
	Yes	No				
[15-25[	13(17,6)	159(92,4)	172	0,24[0,11-0,5]	14,4	0,0002
[25-35[	22(25,6)	64(74,4)	86	Reference		
[35-45[	4(12,1)	29(87,9)	33	0,40[0,12-1,27]	1,8	0,1404
[45-55[	4(20)	16(80)	20	0,73[0,22-2,41]	0,05	0,7756
[55-65[	2(16,7)	10(83,3)	12	0,58[0,11-2,86]	0,09	0,7531
[65-75[	1(11,1)	8(89,9)	9	0,36[0,04-3,07]	0,31	0,4473
[75-85[	0(0)	1(100)	1	Undefined		
Total	**46**	**287**	**333**			

According to Table IV, there was a statically significant association (OR= 0.24[0.11-0.5]; %2 > 3.84 and p < 0.05) only between respondents aged 15-25. For all other age groups, there was no statistically significant association.

Table V. Occupation and use of VCT

Profession	Use of VCT		Total	OR [95% CI]	x2	p-value
	Yes	No				
Trader	4(16)	21(84)	25	0,42[0,13-1,45]	1,2	0,2667
Cultivator	16(30,8)	36(69,2)	52	Reference		
Resourceful	3(6,3)	45(93,8)	48	0,15[0,04-0,56]	8,2	0,0019
Student	6(6,3)	90(93,8)	96	0,15[0,05-0,41]	14,1	0,0001
Teacher	5(26,3)	14(73,7)	19	0,80[0,25-2,61]	0,005	0,7778
Student	3(10,7)	25(89,3)	28	0,27[0,07-1,03]	3,01	0,0558
Civil servant	1(4,8)	20(95,2)	21	0,11[0,01-0,91]	4,3	0,0166
Liberal	2(20)	8(80)	10	0,56[0,11-0,95]	0,1	0,7091
Housekeeper	6(17,6)	28(82,4)	34	0,48[0,17-1,39]	1,2	0,2119
Total	**46**	**287**	**333**			

Table V shows that there is a statistically significant association between occupation and low VCT use, that between occupations: civil servant (OR=0.11[0.01-0.91]), student (OR=0.15[0.05-0.41]) and handyman (OR=0.15[0.04-0.56]); x2and p-value respectively greater than 3.84 and less than 0.05. There was no significant association between other occupations.

Table VI. Marital status and VCT use

Marital status	Use of VCT		Total	OR [95% CI]	x2	p-value
	Yes	No				
Single	21(11,7)	158(88,3)	179	0,22[0,05-1]	2,5	0,0677
Married	22(15,1)	124(84,9)	146	0,3[0,07-1,32]	1,4	0,1215
Widow(er)	3(37,5)	5(62,5)	8	Reference		
Total	**46**	**287**	**333**			

According to the table above, there is no statistically significant association between marital status and low VCT use ($x2 < 3.84$ and $P > 0.05$).

Table VII. Religion and VCT use

Religion	Use of VCT		Total	OR [95% CI]	x2p-value
	Yes	No			
Animist	0(0)	3(100)		3	Undefined
No	2(18,2)	9(81,8)		11	Reference
Christian	40(13,5)	256(86,5)	296	0,70[0,15-3,37]	10,6511
Muslim woman	4(17,4)	19(82,6)	23	0,94[0,14-6,17]	11
Total	**46**	**287**	**333**		

The data shown in Table VII for the association between religion and low VCT use are not statistically significant ($x2 < 3.84$ and $P > 0.05$).

Table VIII. Distribution of respondents by residence and VCT use

Residence (municipality)	Use of VCT		Total	OR [95% CI]	$x2$	p-value
	Yes	No				
Bondoyi	23(20,9)	87(79,1)	110	Reference		
Musadi	11(11)	89(89)	100	0,47[0,22-1,02]	3,1	0,0613
Mwene-Ditu	12(9,8)	111(90,2)	123	0,41[0,19-0,87]	4,82	0,0282
Total	**46**	**287**	**333**			

The table above informs a statistically significant association between the residence and low VCT use (OR= 0.41[0.19-0.87]; %2= 4.82 and p < 0.05) than between the commune of Mwene-Ditu. There was no statistically significant association for any of the other two communes.

Table IX. Distribution of respondents by level of education and use of CDV

Level of education	Use of VCT		Total	OR [95% CI]	$x2$	p-value
	Yes	not				
No	7(63,6)	4(36,4)	11	Reference		
Primary	18(12,4)	127(87,6)	145	0,08[0,02-0,30]	16,3	0,0003
Secondary	13(10,2)	114(89,8)	127	0,05[0,01-0,2]	25	0,0000
Higher education and universities	8(16)	42(84)	50	0,11[0,03-0,46]	8,6	0,0028
Total	**46**	**287**	**333**			

According to Table IX, there is a statistically significant association between level of education and low VCT use, namely: primary (OR=0.08[0.02-0.30]), secondary (OR=0.05[0.01-0.2]) and university (OR=0.11[0.03-0.46]); %2> 3.84.and p< 0.05.

4.2.2. *Associations between information received about HIV infection and use of voluntary HIV counselling and testing (VCT) services*

Table X. Distribution according to knowledge of HIV transmission routes and VCT use

Transmission routes	Use of VCT		Total	OR [95% CI]	x2	p-value
	Yes	No				
Transversal	3(10,7)	25(89,3)	28	0,67[0,19-2,33]	0,13	0,7769
Sanguine	10(11,2)	79(88,8)	89	0,7[0,33-1,49]	0,5	0,4692
Sexual	33(15,3)	183(84,7)	216	Reference		
Total	**46**	**287**	**333**			

From the table above, it can be seen that there is no statistically significant association between knowledge of transmission routes and low VCT use ($x2<3.84$ at ddl =1 and p-value >0.05).

Table XI. Distribution of interviewees according to knowledge of HIV prevention methods and use of VCT

Means of prevention	Use of VCT		Total	OR [95% CI]	x2	p-value
	Yes	No				
ABC	35(15,6)	190(84,4)	225	Reference		
Avoid sharp objects	7(9,2)	69(90,8)	76	0,55[0,23-1,3]	1,4	0,1858
PMTCT	2(14,3)	12(85,7)	14	0,9[0,19-4,22]	0,06	1
Transfusion safety	2(13,8)	16(86,2)	18	0,68[0,15-3,08]	0,03	1
Total	**46**	**287**	**333**			

According to Table XII, there is no statistically significant association between knowledge of HIV prevention methods and low VCT use: %2 and p-value less than 3.84 at ddl =1 and greater than 0.05 respectively.

Table XII. Distribution by source of information on HIV and use of CDV

Source of information	Use of VCT		Total	OR [CI at 95%]	x2	p-value
	Yes	No				
Friend and family	4(16)	21(84)	25	0,13[0,04-0,46]	10	0,0007
School/University	17(6,6)	240(93,4)	257	0,05[0,02-0,11]	74	0,0000
Radio	2(16,7)	10(83,3)	12	0,14[0,03-0,71]	5,03	0,0181
Structure of health	22(59,5)	15(40,5)	35	Reference		
Television	1(50)	1(50)	2	0,68[0,04-11,8]	0,2	1
Total	**46**	**287**	**333**			

From the table above, there is a statistically significant association between the source of information and low VCT use: (x2> 3.84 and p< 0.05 at dll 1) than between the following sources: friend and family, school/university and radio. And no statistically significant associations were reported for all other sources.

4.2.3. *Associations between knowledge about VCT and its use*

Table XIII. Distribution of cases according to knowledge of screening location and use of VCT

Knowledge of the place	Use of VCT		Total	OR [95% CI]	x2	p-value
	Yes	No				
Yes	42(17,6)	196(82,4)	238		Reference	
No	4(4,2)	140(95,8)	95	0,21[0,07-0,59]	9,2	0,0007
Total	**46**	**287**	**333**			

According to the data repeated in the table XIII, it is apparent that there is association statistically significant between not knowing where to get HIV testing and low VCT use (OR =0.21[0.07-0.59]; x2>3.84 and p<0.05 at ddl 1).

Table XIV. Distribution of respondents according to knowledge of the importance of testing and use of VCT

Importance of screening	Use of VCT		otal	OR [95% CI]	x2	p-value
	Yes	No				
Yes	45(14,2)	271(85,8)	316	Reference		
No	1(5,9)	16(94,1)	17	0,38[0,05-2,91]	0,4	0,4852
Total	**46**	**287**	**333**			

It emerges of the table of contingent above that there is no not of association statistically significant between knowledge of the importance of screening and low VCT use: %2 less than 3.84 at ddl 1 and p-value greater than 0.05.

Table XV. Distribution according to awareness and use of VCT

Awareness raising received	Use of VCT		Total	OR [95% CI]	x2	p-value
	Yes	No				
Yes	39(22)	138(78)	177	Reference		
No	7(4,5)	149(95,5)	156	0,16[0,07-0,38]	20	0,0000
Total	**46**	**287**	**333**			

Table XV shows that there is a statistically significant association between lack of awareness of screening and low VCT use (%2 > 3.84 at ddl 1 and p-value < 0.05).

Table XVI. Distribution of respondents according to knowledge of when to test for HIV and use of VCT

Moments	Use of VCT		Total	OR [95% CI]	x2	p-value
	Yes	No				
At any time	6(14,6)	35(85,4)	41	0,61[0,23-1,63]	0,58	0,3659
In case of injury	10(14,5)	59(85,5)	69	0,60[0,27-1,36]	1,05	0,2426
In case of illness	7(5,9)	111(94,1)	118	0,22[0,09-0,55]	10,8	0,0006
In case of violence sexual	23(21,9)	82(78,1)	105	Reference		
Total	**46**	**287**	**333**			

From XVI's table, it appears that there is a statistically significant association between knowledge of when to test for HIV and low VCT use ($\%2 > 3.84$ at ddl 1 and p-value less than 0.05) in case of illness only and no statistically significant association between other times of testing.

4.2.4. Association between attitude towards the HIV status of the relative and the use of voluntary HIV testing centres (VCT)

Table XVII. Distribution of cases according to the attitude towards the HIV status of the and the use of VCT

Attitude	Use of VCT		Total	OR [95% CI]	x2	p-value
	Yes	No				
Continuing to live together	13(10,7)	109(89,3)	122	0,64[0,32-1,27]	1,2	0,249
Making a separation	33(15,6)	178(84,4)	211	Reference		
Total	**46**	**287**	**333**			

The table above shows that there is no statistically significant association between attitude towards the relative's HIV status and low VCT use: chi-square less than 3.84 at ddl =1 and p-value greater than 0.05.

Chapter 5

DISCUSSION

Our study focused on the factors that explain the low use of voluntary counselling and testing (VCT) services for HIV infection by the adult population. To this end, 333 statistical units were surveyed in the town of Mwene-Ditu, Lomami province in the DRC.

The objectives of this study were to identify the socio-demographic characteristics of VCT users and to determine the factors associated with low use by the population aged 15 years and over.

The gender distribution reveals that men had low utilization of VCT services at 13.6% compared to women at 14%. However, this small difference observed is not statistically significant as the p-value is greater than 0.05 and the calculated chi-square is at the theoretical one of 3.84 at the degree of freedom (ddl) of 1. The hypothesis that gender should be a factor in the low use of VCT in our study was refuted. This fact observed in our study would be related to other factors.

Men's use of VCT was low in our study. This reflects their limited access to health services. In Uganda, the analysis by Larsson et al. (2010).from 2008 to 2009 showed the same situation found in our study, as men were not using HIV testing services. Hutchinson (2006) showed the opposite situation to that shown in our study. In his study on the voluntary use of HIV testing services in the Eastern Cape, the result showed that men were more likely to use voluntary HIV testing services than women. This low VCT uptake by men observed in our study is sometimes said to be due to the fear of positive test results.

Despite the fact that women used VCT, 14% in our study; this result is still lower than those found by Peltzer (2009) and Snow (2010) in their studies, where they showed that women had more access to VCT than men. Women accounted for 65%. This situation is similar in Burkina Faso, where the study by Sarker et al (2009) showed good uptake of screening services by women. The low proportion of women who used VCT services observed in our study is sometimes attributed to sample fluctuation.

The significant proportion of adults in the town of Mwene-Ditu, 86%, as shown in our study, have never been tested for HIV. This situation would be linked to the lack of intensified sensitisation on screening targeting the adult population in general; whereas ignorance of serological status has been shown to be an important factor in the spread of the disease (Kitahata et al., 2009). This idea is shared by Rozebaum (2010), as more than 70% of sexual infections come from people who do not know their HIV status. However, testing remains the best entry point for HIV prevention (Memmi et al., 2010).

The proportion of people who do not know their HIV status is very high in our study. This situation is far from achieving the Sustainable Development Goals, in which one of the major objectives in relation to the fight against HIV infection is that the proportion of people who know their HIV status reaches 90%. Intensified awareness of adult testing is needed to increase the proportion of people who know their HIV status.

People in the 15-25 age group were more represented in our study (51.7%) compared to 0.3% in the 75-85 age group. The average age of the respondents was estimated at 28.6 (Sdv 13) and 75% of the respondents were under 35 years old. As we can see, young people were more represented because during the period of our survey, they were more likely to be found in households at the time of the survey. This period was also characterised by containment as one of the preventive measures against the coronavirus pandemic decreed by the Congolese government to limit the spread of this new virus.

Young age (15-25 years) was a factor in the low use of VCT in our study, with a p-value of less than 0.05. In this respect, our hypothesis was confirmed as we demonstrated in our introductory section.

Our analyses found that young age was a factor in low VCT uptake. The same situation has been demonstrated in Botswana, where sexually active young people (under 25 years of age) were not willing to be tested for HIV (Fako et al., 2006). The same was found by Peltzer et al, (2009) and Johnston et al, (2010) in their study, according to which young people under the age of 25 were less likely to know their HIV status.

This demonstrated situation could be explained by the fact that there are barriers that hinder adolescents' access to voluntary HIV counselling and testing, including: parental consent requirements, fear of a positive result and stigma, reactions of relatives and negative attitudes of health care providers or lack of confidentiality.

In our series, farmers represented the largest proportion of people who had ever been tested for HIV voluntarily (30.8%).

State officials (4.8%), students and resourceful people (6.3%) made low use of VCT. The associations between the occupations: students, government employees and resourceful people significantly influence the low use of VCT, as the p-value is less than 0.05 and the chi-square is greater than 3.84 at ddl = 1.

As we can see in our study, the occupation of the farmers would be a factor in the low use of VCT because it is the main occupation in the area. In this respect, our study would be confronted with a sampling bias, due to the fact that during the survey, many of the farmers were in the fields, occupied with rural activities. This justifies their low representativeness in our study. This result does not corroborate the one found by Mbompi-Keou et al. (2013) where it was shown that students represented the majority of people who had already been tested, more than half of them, i.e. 52%. This observation in our study would be linked to the non-permanent awareness or insufficient number of advertising signs (awareness) relating to testing in the workplace and schools.

Our study showed that widows and widowers used HIV testing and counselling more (37.5%) compared to married and single people at 15.1% and 11.7% respectively. The association between marital status and low HIV VCT uptake was not significant, as the p-value was greater than 0.05. The observed low uptake is thought to be related to other factors.

With regard to religion, respondents with no religious affiliation used the VCT service (18.2%) compared to 0% of animist respondents. However, the association between religion and low VCT use is not statistically significant, as the p-value is greater than 0.05.

Thus, the hypothesis that religion is a factor in the low use of voluntary HIV counselling and testing services is not confirmed in this series. This situation of low use is linked to the low representation of certain religions in our environment.

According to residence, 20.9% of respondents in the commune of Bondoyi used VCT, compared with 11% and 9.8% in the other communes of Musadi and Mwene-Ditu respectively. The association between respondents in the commune of Mwene-Ditu and low VCT use is statistically significant (p-value less than 0.05 and chi-square greater than 3.84). We note that respondents in the communes of Bondoyi and Musadi used VCT more than those in Mwene-Ditu. This fact would be justified by the fact that there are not many educated people in the previous communes who are not afraid of knowing their serological status, unlike those in the commune of Mwene-Ditu, which is an advanced and urban commune where people can have risky behaviour.

Educated respondents at all levels of education (primary, secondary and university) had a low use of VCT at 12.4%, 10.2% and 16% respectively, compared to 63.6% of respondents with no education. The association between the level of education and the low use of VCT is statistically significant, p-value less than 0.05 and Chi-square greater than 3.84, at ddl=1. This confirms our hypothesis. This result is similar to that found in the study conducted by Mwembo et al. (2012), according to which low level of education was a factor determining ignorance of HIV status among women.

This situation is justified by the fact that the awareness messages through the panels relating to screening in primary, secondary and university educational institutions are not only permanent but also insufficient in our environment to reinforce the awareness messages on VCT.

Respondents who knew the transmissible and blood-borne routes of HIV transmission had low VCT use at 10.7% and 11.2% compared to 15.3% of respondents who knew the sexual route. However, the association between knowledge of HIV transmission routes and low VCT use was not statistically significant (p-value greater than 0.05).

A similar study showed that people who had a good level of information about modes of HIV transmission were more likely to accept HIV testing (Fylkesnes et al. (Fylkesnes et al., 2004; Degraft et al., 2005, Peltzer et al., 2009).

Concerning the source of information about HIV testing, it appears that respondents informed about HIV through school and university, friends, family and radio made little use of VCT, respectively at 6.6% and 16% and 16.7%, compared to 59.5% of those who were informed through health facilities. There is a significant association between the sources of information (school/university, friend and family and radio) and low VCT use, p-value less than 0.05. This would be related to the quality of the information disseminated.

After analysis and interpretation of the data collected in our study, it appears that a low proportion of adults in the town of Mwene-Ditu knew their HIV status (14%), due to various factors, including stigma, discrimination, fear of positive results, etc. This proportion found in our study (14%) is higher than that found in France, where the proportion of the population with knowledge of HIV status was estimated at 8% (Girard et al., 2008). This proportion found in our study (14%), is higher than that found in France where the proportion of the population with knowledge of HIV status was estimated at 8% (Girard et al., 2008).

However, the result of 14% found in our study is lower than that found by Mbompi-keou et al. (2013) where 76.2% of participants had knowledge of their HIV status. This observed difference would be related to the attitudes and opinions of each population but also to their social and demographic characteristics on the one hand and to the sample size on the other.

The reasons given for refusing to undergo voluntary HIV testing included: fear of discrimination, stigmatisation, fear of a positive result, and indiscretion or lack of confidentiality on the part of health care providers. Thus, we find that the hypothesis put forward in our study has been confirmed. This is similar to the situation found in the studies by Meiberg et al,

(2008) Makhlouf et al. (2009); Neuman et al, (2013) and Maman et al. (2009), which found that fear of stigma led to fear and reluctance to test for HIV. Stigma and fear of a positive test result were also reasons for refusal of voluntary HIV testing in Uganda (Larsson et al., 2010; Meiberg et al., 2008; Mutalemwa et al., 2008; Kranzer et al., 2008; Osinde et al., 2011).

Apart from the other factors identified in this study that explain a low proportion of VCT users, ignorance of where to get tested was also one of the factors in the low uptake of VCT in our study. However, it was demonstrated in our study that ignorance of the place of testing would be one of the factors in the low use of voluntary HIV counselling and testing services. To this end, our hypothesis is affirmed. This would be justified by the lack of or low mass awareness regarding voluntary HIV testing in the town of Mwene-Ditu.

CONCLUSION

HIV/AIDS infection is one of the most devastating communicable diseases of the last three decades. The modern world still faces serious multi-faceted epidemics, with ignorance of HIV status being a major factor in the spread of the disease.

To do this, we conducted a cross-sectional and analytical study from 15 June to 15 July 2020 in the town of Mwene-Ditu. It consisted of identifying the socio-demographic characteristics of people who used the VCT service, and also determining the factors that explain the low use of this service by this population.

Males; people under 45 years of age; government officials; students and resourceful people; singles; Christians; residents of the commune of Mwene-Ditu; and those with primary and secondary education made low use of VCT.

The factors that explain the low use of VCT were: age, occupation, level of education, residence, source of information on HIV, lack of knowledge of where to go for testing, lack of awareness of testing and lack of information on when to go for HIV testing.

Discrimination was one of the main reasons why people in Mwene-Ditu refused to be tested for HIV.

The use of VCT is still a challenge in the adult population of the town of Mwene-Ditu because the results of our survey showed a low proportion of users due to several factors, such as: age under 35 years, occupation category, low level of education, ignorance of the place of testing, to mention only those. Intensifying awareness of voluntary HIV testing would be necessary to increase the proportion of people who know their HIV status.

Conflicts of interest: We declare no conflicts of interest.

BIBLIOGRAPHIC REFERENCES

-I- Agudu S, Nadia A, Falayan B, Marenike O, Ezeanolue E, Echezona E (2016). *Seeking Wilder acces to HIV testing for adolescents in sub-saharan africa. Pediatric research,*
79(6):838-845.

-I- Anon (2014). *Guidelines on Post Exposure Prophylaxis for HIV. Recommandations for a Public Heath Approach. OMS, Genève, pp 34.*

4- ASPC (2006). *HIV testing and counselling: policy in transition, Toronto, PHAC, pp 53.*

-I- Degraft J, Paz VS, Kasote A, Tsui A (2005). *HIV voluntary counseling and testing service preferences in a rural Malawi population. AIDS Behav, 9(4): 475-84.*

I- Desclaux A, Ky-zerbo O, Somé SF, Manklouf OC (2014). *The campaigns Community-based HIV testing promotion in West Africa: user perceptions in Burkina Faso. NIH-PA Author Manuscript, 21(4):57-65.*

-I- Fako TT (2006). *Social and psychological factors associatited with willingness to test for HIV infection among Young people in Botswana. AIDS care, 18(3): 201-7.*

-I- Fylkesnes K, Siziya S (2004). *A randomized trial acceptability of voluntary HIV counseling and testing. Top Med in Health, 9(5): 566-572.*

-I- Hansoti B, Hill SE, Whalen M (2017). *Patient and provider attitudes to emergency department based HIV counseling and in South Africa. S Afr J HIV Med. 18(1): 707. http://doi.org/10.4102/sajhivmed.v18i1.707.*

-I- Hejoaka F (2009). *Care and secrecy: Being a mother of children living with HIV in Burkina-Faso, social science et Medecine, 69(6): 869-876.*

-I- *Hutchinson PL, Mahlalela X (2006). Utilization of voluntary counseling and testing services in the Eastern cape, South Africa. AIDS Care, 18(5):446-55.*

I- Girad PM, Cazein F, Pilonel J, Le strat Y, Lot F et al. (2008). *HIV-AIDS infection in France Institut de veille sanitaire. Numéro thématique. BEH, (45-46): 433-60.*

I- Johnston L, O'bra H, Chapra M, Mathews C, Townsend L, Sabin K et al. (2010). *The association of voluntary counseling and testing acceptance and perceived likelihood of being HIV-infected among men with multiple sex parteners in South African township. AIDSBehav., 14(4): 922-31.*

I- Kitahata MM, Gange SJ, Abraham AG, Merriman B, Saag MS, Justice AC et al.

(2009) . *Effect of versus deferred antiretroviral therapy for HIV on survival. N Engl J Med. 360(18): 1815-1826.*

-I- Kranzer K, Mcgrath N, Saul J, Crampin AC, Jahn A, Malema S et coll. (2008). *Individual, household and community factors associated with HIV test refusal in rural Malawi. Trop Med Int Health, 13(11):1341-50.doi:10.1111/j.1365-3156.200802148.X.Epub 2008. Oct 6.*

I- Larson EC, Thorson A, Nsabagasani X, Namusoko S, Popenoe R, Ekstrom AM (2010) . *Mistrust in mariage-reasons why men do not accept couple HIV testing during antenatal care-a qualitative study in eastern Uganda. BMC Public Heath, 10(1):1-9*

I- Lingani S, Korbéogo G (2015). *HIV/AIDS as an accident in the course of a lifetime: slow discovery, social management and exclusion of HIV-positive women in Burkina - Faso. Recherches féministes, 28(2):243-264. http//doi.org/10.7202/1034184ar*

-I- Maklouf OC, Bott S, Carrière P, Parsons M, Pulerwitz S, Gutenberg N et coll. (2009). *HIV testing, treatement and prevention: genetic Tools for operational research, World Health Organization, Geneva, pp 66.*

-b Maman S, Ablet L, Paker L, Lane T, Chirowodza A, Ntogwisangu J et coll. (2009). *A comparison of VIH stigma and discrimination in five international sites: the influence of care and treatement resources in high prevalence settings. Socsci Med. 68(12): 2271-8.*

-I- Marks G, Crepaz N, Janssen RS (2006). *Estimating sexual transmission of HIV from persons aware and unaware that they are infected with the virus in the USA. AIDS, 20(10): 1447-50.*

-I- Marks G, crepaz N, Senterfitt JW, Janssen RS (2005). *Meta-analysis of high-risk sexual behavior in persons are and unaware they are infected with HIV in the States. Implications for HIV prevention programs. J cquir Immune Decsyndr, 39(4): 446-53.*

-b Mbopi-keou FX, Kalla GCM, Tchouamani H, Deugoue C, Mbahe S, Angwafo III F et coll. (2007). *Effectiveness of mobile units for mass HIV testing in sub-Saharan Africa:the Cameroon pioneer experience. Health sc Dis. 8(4):18-21.*

I- Mbopi-keou FX, Nguefack TG, Kalla GCM, Viche L, Noubom M (2013). *Epidemiological profile of HIV infection during an awareness campaign in Yaoundé, Cameroon. Pamj, 15: 119. Doi: 10.11604/pamj.2013.15.119.2968*

-I- Meiberg AE, Bos A, Onya HE, Schaalma HP (2008). *Fear of stigmatization as barrier to voluntary HIV counseiling and testing in South Africa. East Afr J Public Heath, 5(2):49-54.*

I- Memmi S, Desgrées du Loû A, Orne G, liemann J, (2010). *HIV/AIDS prevention strategies in low- and middle-income countries. Workingpaper of CEPED, Paris: Université Paris Descartes, INED, IRD, pp 78*

-I- Mutalemwa P, Kisoka W, Nyigo V, Barongo V, Malecela MN, Kisinza WN (2008). *Manifestations and reduction strategies of stigma and discrimination on people living with HIV/AIDS in Tanzania. Tanzan JHeaith Res, 10(4): 220-5.*

I- Mwembo TA, Kalenga MPK, Donnen P, Chenge MF, Humblet P, Dramaix M et al. *(2012).Deliveries with unknown HIV status in Lubumbashi, DR Congo: proportion and determinants. Panafrican-med-journal 12:25. http://www.panafrican- med-journal.com/content/article/12/25/full/*

-I- Neuman M, Obermeyer CM, Desclaux A, Wanyenze R, Ky-zerbo O, Cherutich P et coll. (2013). *For the MATCH study group experiences of stigma, discrimination, care and support a mongpeople living, with HIV: A four country study. AIDS Behav. 17(5): 1796-808.*

-I- Obemeyer CM, Sankara A, Bastien V, Parsons M (2009). *Gender and HIV testing in Burkina-Faso: an exploratory study. Soc SciMed., 69(6): 877-84.*

-I-WHO (2016). *Sixty-ninth World Health Assembly, Draft global health sector strategies for HIV, 2016-202, Geneva, WHO, pp.52*

-I-WHO (2019). *Key HIV benchmarks 2018, Geneva, WHO, pp37.*

WHO. (2017). *HIV/AIDS; Fact sheet updated November 2017, Geneva, WHO, pp 38*

UNAIDS (2019). *World AIDS Day 2019 Fact Sheet, Global HIV Statistics 2109, New York, UNAIDS, pp 7.*

-I- Osinde MO, Kaye DK, Kakoire O (2011). *Intimate Partner violence among women with HIV infection in rural Uganda: critical implications for Policy and practice. BMC Wome's Heath, 11(1):50-61.*

-I- Peltezer K, Matseke G, Mzolo T, Majaja M (2009). *Determinants of knowledge of HIV status in South Africa: results from a population-based HIV survery. BMC Public Health, 9(1): 174-83.*

-I- PNLS (2017). *Guide de prise en charge intégrée du VIH en République Démocratique du Congo 2017, Kinshasa, PNLS, pp 130.*

-I- NLSP (2020). *Annual Report 2019 BPC, Lomami, PNLS, pp 37.*

-I- PNMLS (2018). *Plan stratégique national de la riposte au VIH/SIDA 2018-2021, Kinshasa, PNMLS, pp 54.*

L PNMLS (2019). *JMS 2018 Report, Kinshasa, PNMLS, pp 72.*

-I- Pulerwitz J, Michaelis A, Weiss E, Lisane B, Mahendra V(2010). *Reducing HIV-Related stigma: Lessons learned from Horizons research and programs. Public Heath reports, 125(2):272-281.*

L Rouamba OK(2016). *Issues and limitations of HIV counselling and testing (VCT) in a low prevalence country in sub-Saharan Africa: the case of Burkina- Faso. Human medicine and pathology. University of Montpellier, French. NNT: 2016MONTTO35tel- 01514386.*

I- Rozenbaum W (2010). *Screening and new prevention strategies for HIV infection. Expert Report 2010. Paris: Haute autorité de santé, pp56.*

-I- Sarker M; Papay J, Traore S, Neuhann F (2009). *Insights on HIV pré-test counseiling following scaling up of PMTCTprogram in rural Heath pots, Burkina-Faso. East Afr J Public Heath.6 (3):280-845.*

-I- Singo A, Assetina K (2016). *Feasibility and acceptability of pediatric HIV care finding in Health setting in Togo. NIH-PA Author Manuscript, 34(2): 76-9.*

-I- Snow RC, Madalane M, Poulsen M (2010). *Are men testing? Sex differentials in HIV testing in Mpumalanga province, South Africa. AIDS Care, 22(9):1060-5.doi: 10.1080/09540/2090319364/.*

-I- Some EN, Meda N (2015). *Does the national program of prevention of mother to Child transmission of HIV (PMTCT) reach it target in Ouagadougou, Burkina-Faso. Afr Heath Sci., 14(4):889-898.*

I- Somé JF, Desclaux A, Ky-zerbo O, Lougué M, Kéré S, Obermeyer C et al. (2014). *HIV testing campaigns, an effective strategy for universal access to prevention and treatment. L 'experience du Burkina-Faso. NIH Public Access Author Manuscript, 24(1):73-79.*

-b *Tshikwej ND, Mukuku O, Kaj MF, Numbi LO, Sakatolo KJB, Okitotsho WS (2017). Seroprevalence and factors associated with acceptance of voluntary HIV counselling and testing in children in Lubumbashi, Democratic Republic of Congo. Pamj 28:82.doi: 10.11604/pamj.2107.28.82.9566.*

-b Tshikwej ND, Mukuku O, Mudekereza R, Karaj E, Bwana EFO, Numbi LO et al. (2015). *Study of risk factors for mother-to-child transmission of HIV in the <<option A>> strategy in Lubumbashi, Democratic Republic of Congo.*

Panafrican-med-journal 22:18. Doi: 10.11604/pamj.2015.22.18.7480.

-I- UNAIDS (2015). *Treatment. Available at :*
http://eprints.kmu.ac.ir/7875/1/JC2484 treatment

4- UNAIDS (2016). *90_90_90_Progress_Reportfmal. Available at:*
*http://www.cfenet.ubc.ca/sites/default/files/uploads/IAS2016/90_90_90_Progress_*
Rep ortFINAL

4-http://www.unicef.org/publications/files/Opportunity_in_Crisis-
Report_EN_052711.pdf

-I- UNICEF/UNAIDS (2017). *Accelerating the pace towards an AIDS-free generation*
in West and Central Africa, UNICEF West and Central Africa Regional Office and
UNAIDS West and Central Africa Regional Support Team 2017, Dakar,
UNICEF/UNAIDS, pp 76.

-I- Van kestern NM, Hospers HJ, Kok G (2007). *Sexual risk behavior armong -*
HIVpositive men who have sex with men: a literature review. Patient Educ Couns,
65(1):5-20.

-I- WHO (2008). *Towards universal access: scaling up priority HIV/AIDS interventions*
in the health sector. Progress Report .Consulté en ligne le 15 Janvier 2020

-I- WHO (2015). *Consolidated guidelines on HIV testing services: 5cs: consent,*
confidentiality, counselling, correct results and connection. Consulté en ligne le 15
Janvier 2020

TABLE OF CONTENTS

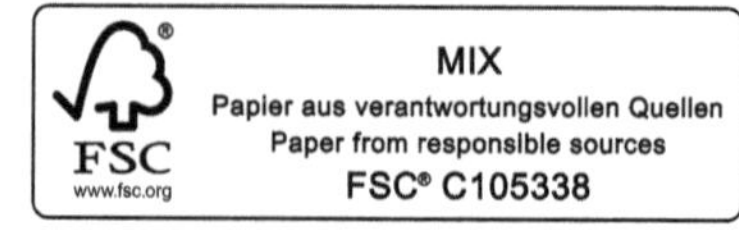

Printed by Books on Demand GmbH, Norderstedt / Germany